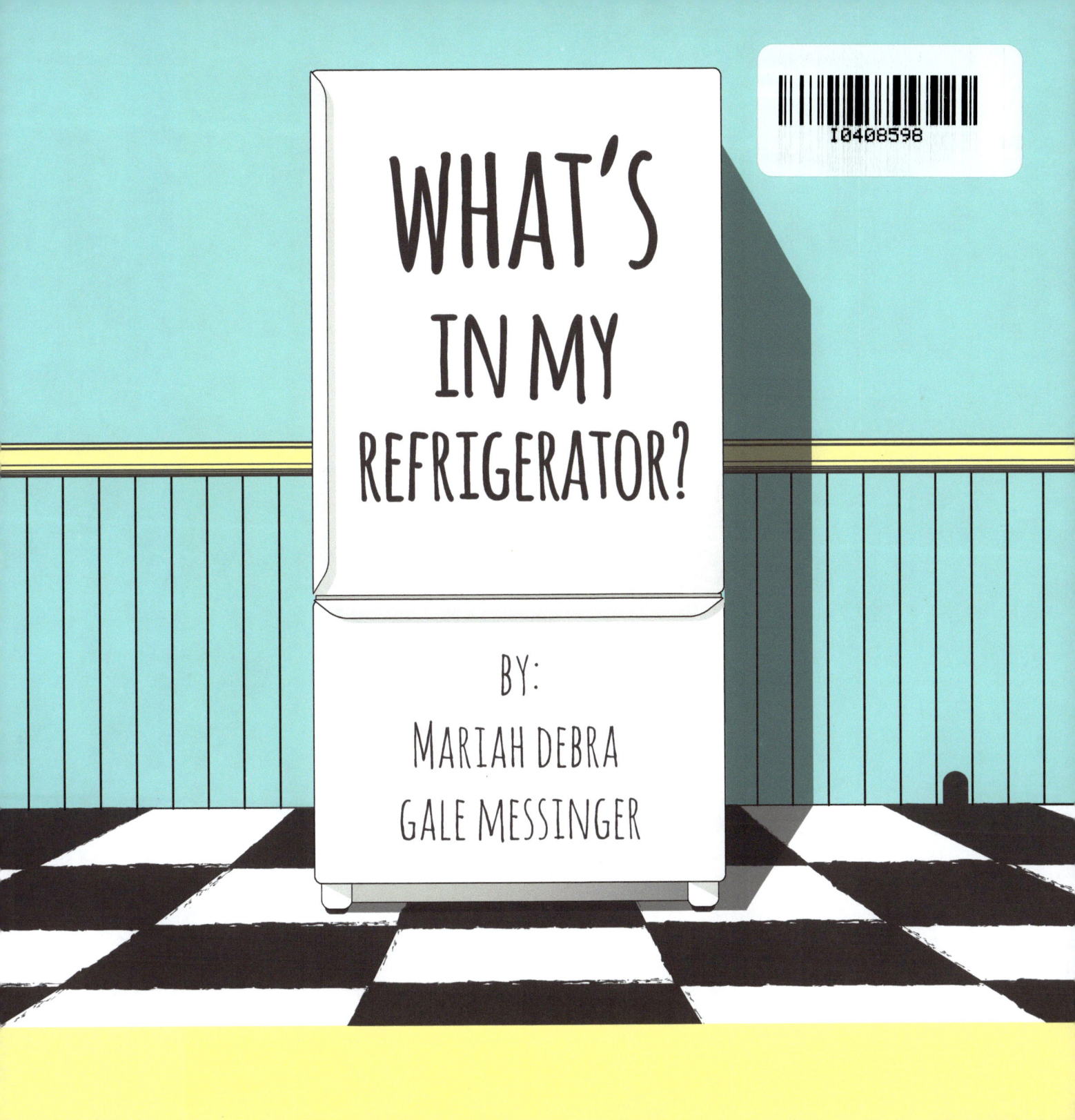

WHAT'S IN MY REFRIGERATOR?

BY:

MARIAH DEBRA

GALE MESSINGER

I0408598

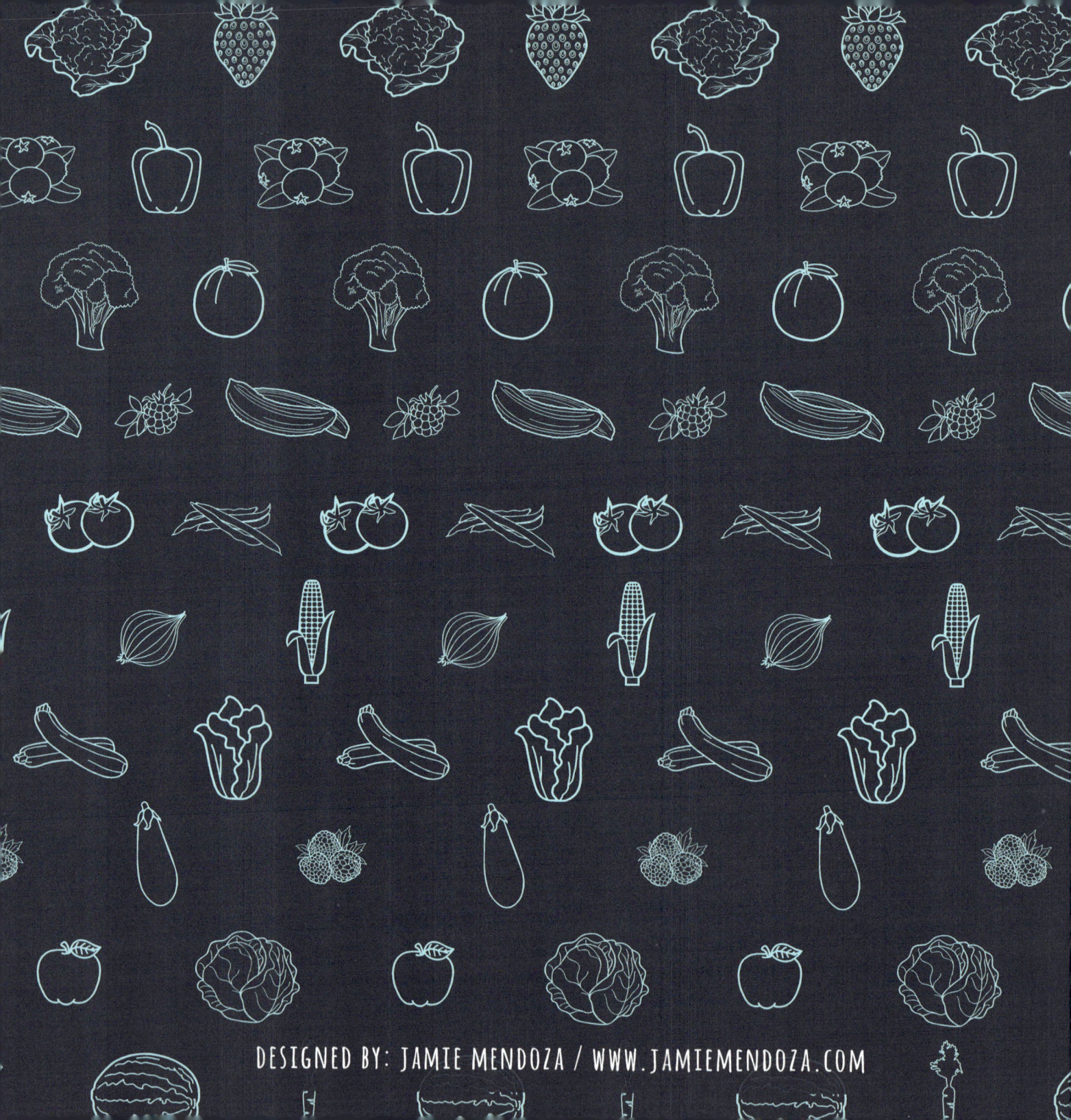

DESIGNED BY: JAMIE MENDOZA / WWW.JAMIEMENDOZA.COM

DEDICATED TO ALL KIDS
AT FOUNDATIONS HOME DAY CARE
PAST AND PRESENT,
WHO LIVE A HEALTHY LIFESTYLE
AND
EAT THEIR COLORS EVERY DAY !

I AM HUNGRY !

I WONDER WHAT'S IN MY REFRIGERATOR?

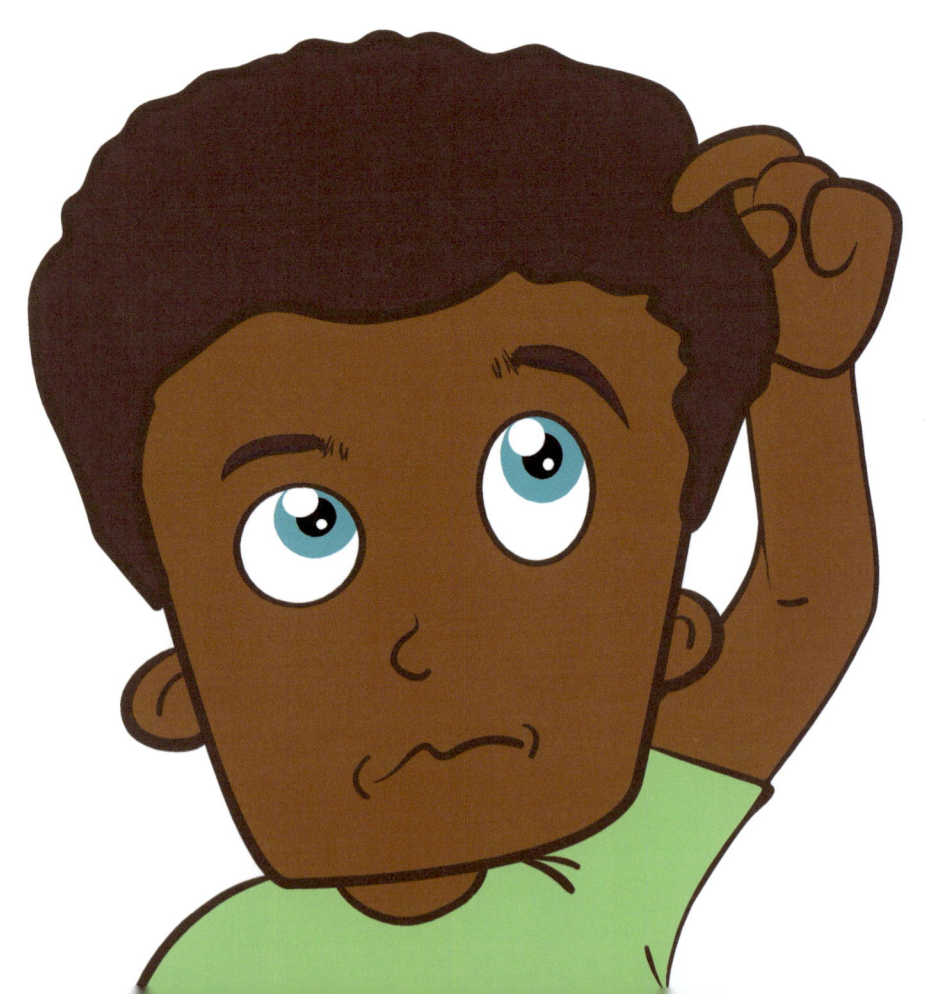

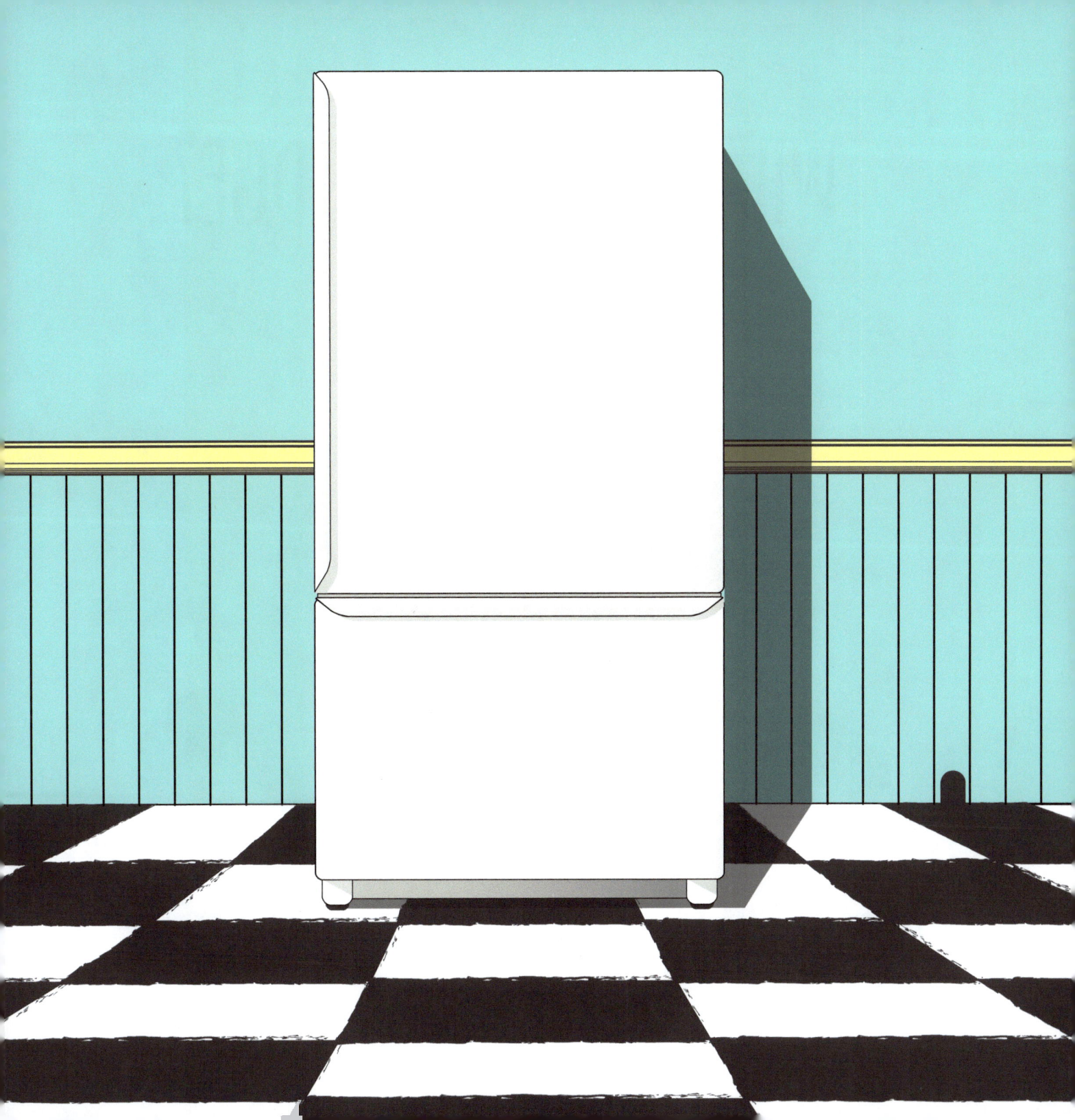

WHAT'S IN MY FRIDGE?

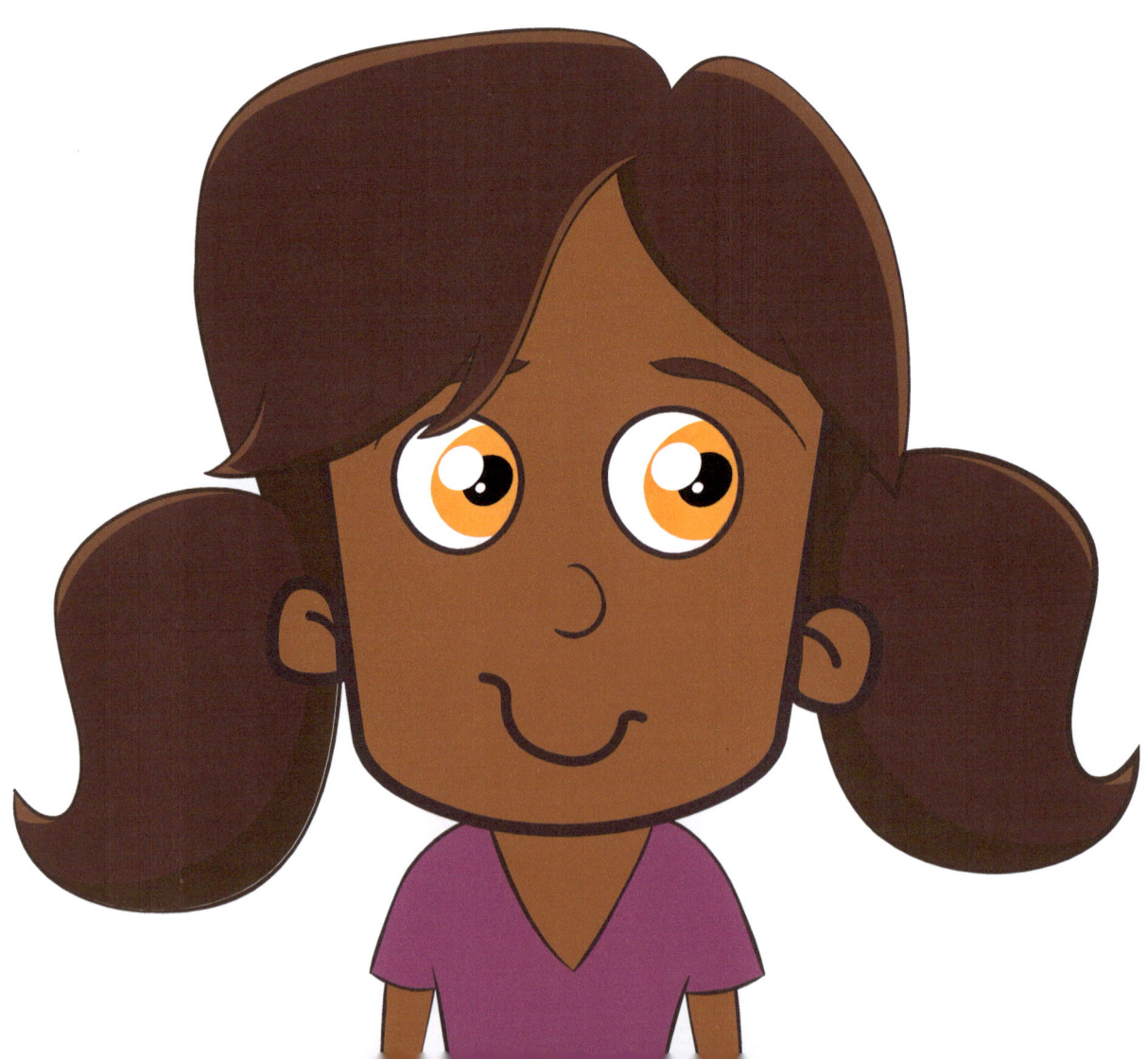

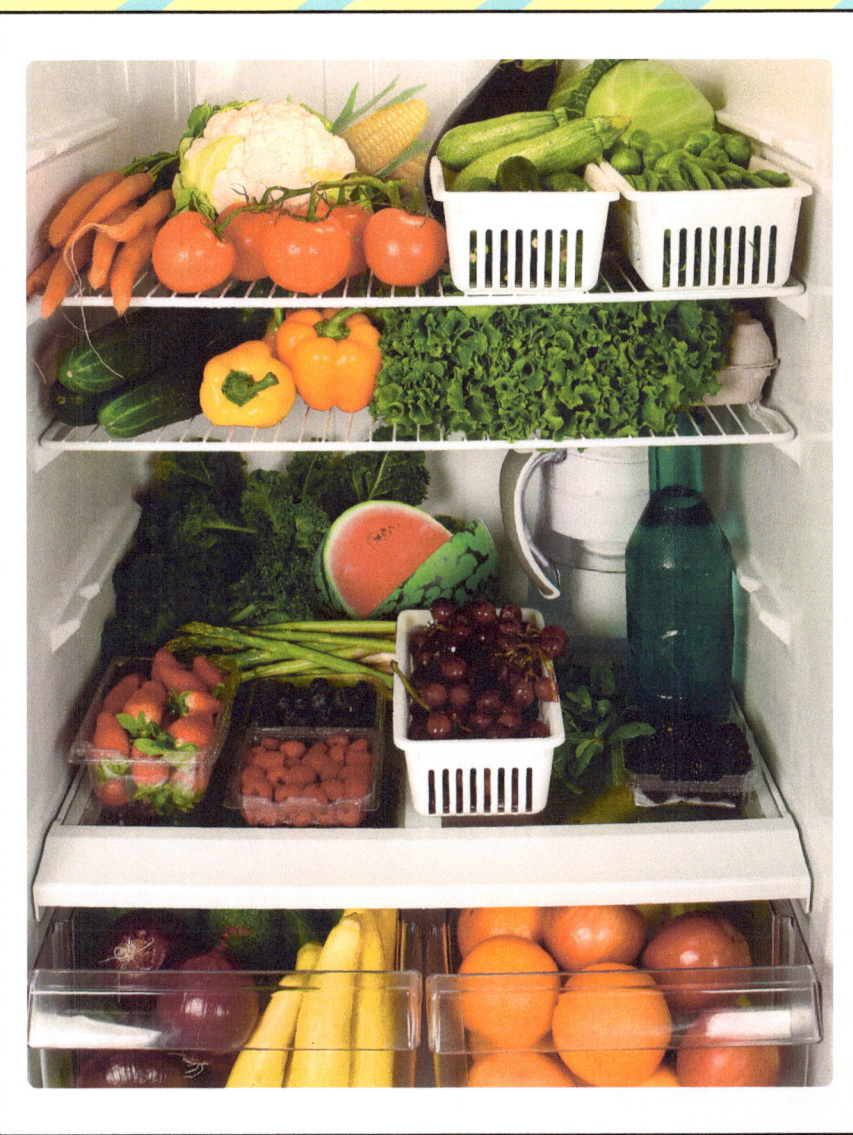

Fresh fruits and vegetables,

All you can eat.

Now, that's what I call

A DELICIOUS TREAT!

Look at the colors!
Every one you can see!
THEY ARE GOOD FOR MY BODY,
My soul and for me!

THEY WILL NOURISH MY ORGANS,

My blood and each cell
With minerals and vitamins,
Enough to keep me well.

THERE ARE...

PURPLE

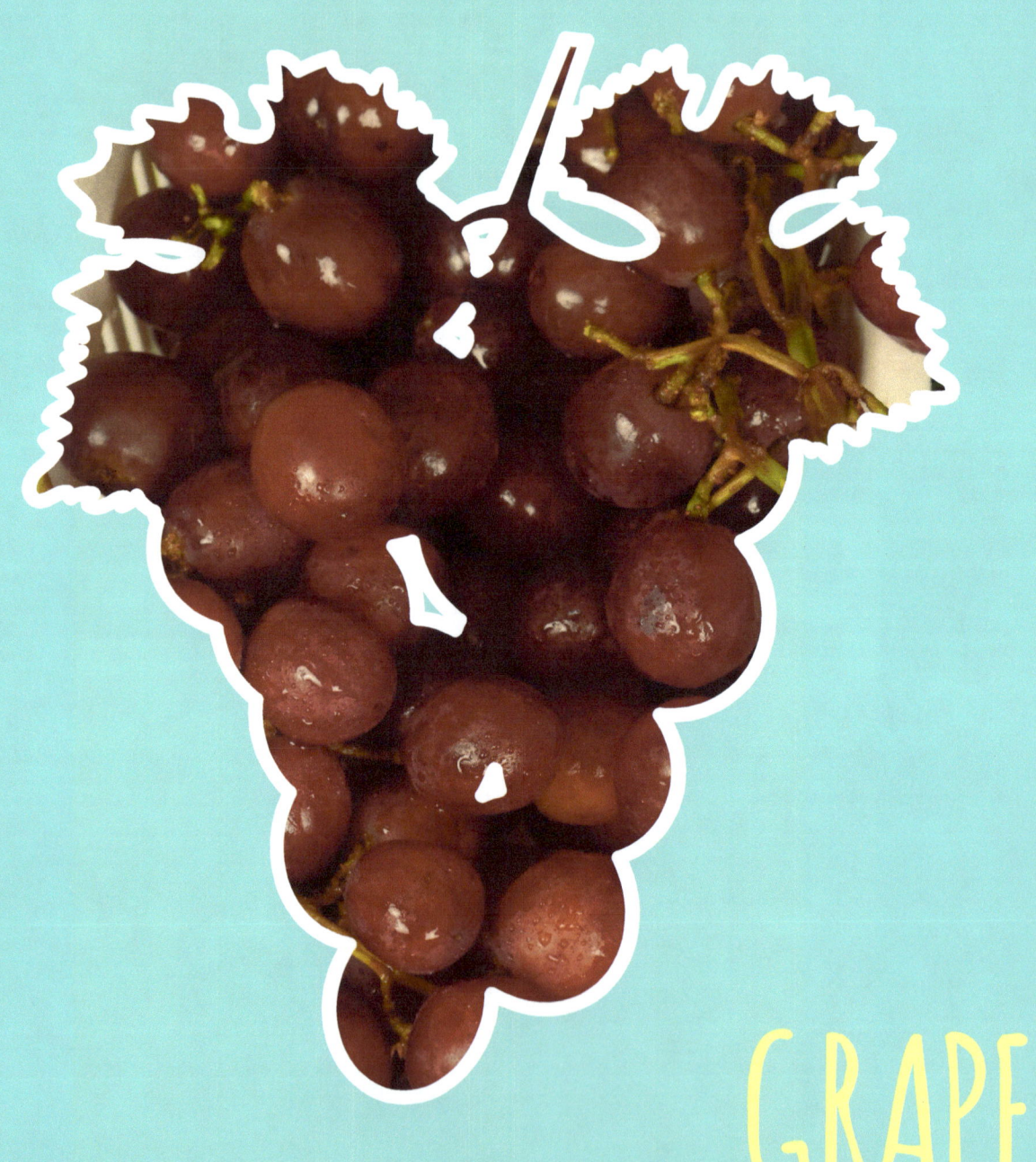

GRAPES

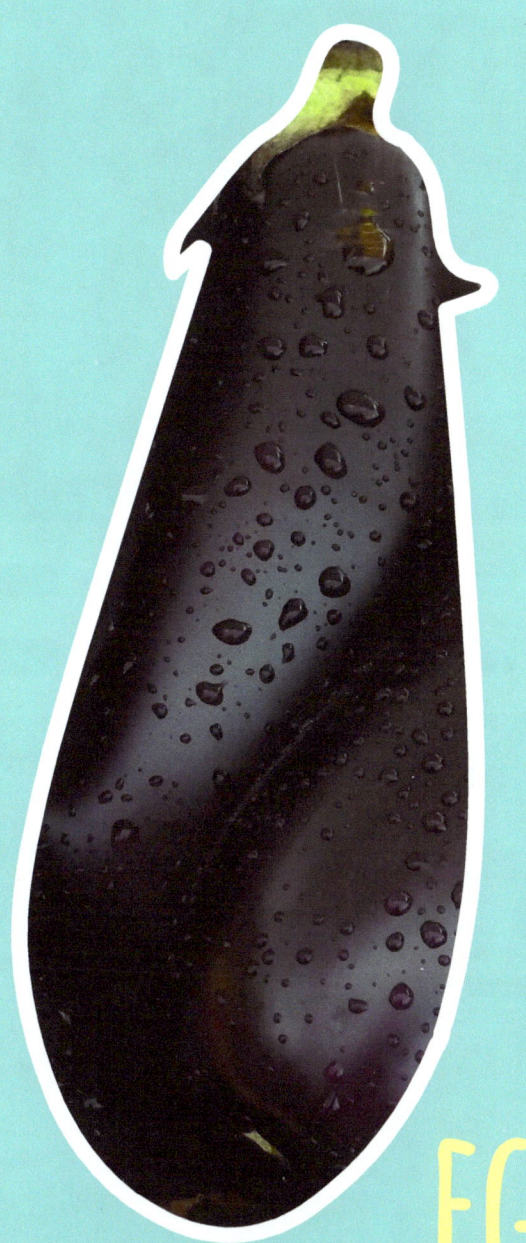

EGGPLANT

BLUE

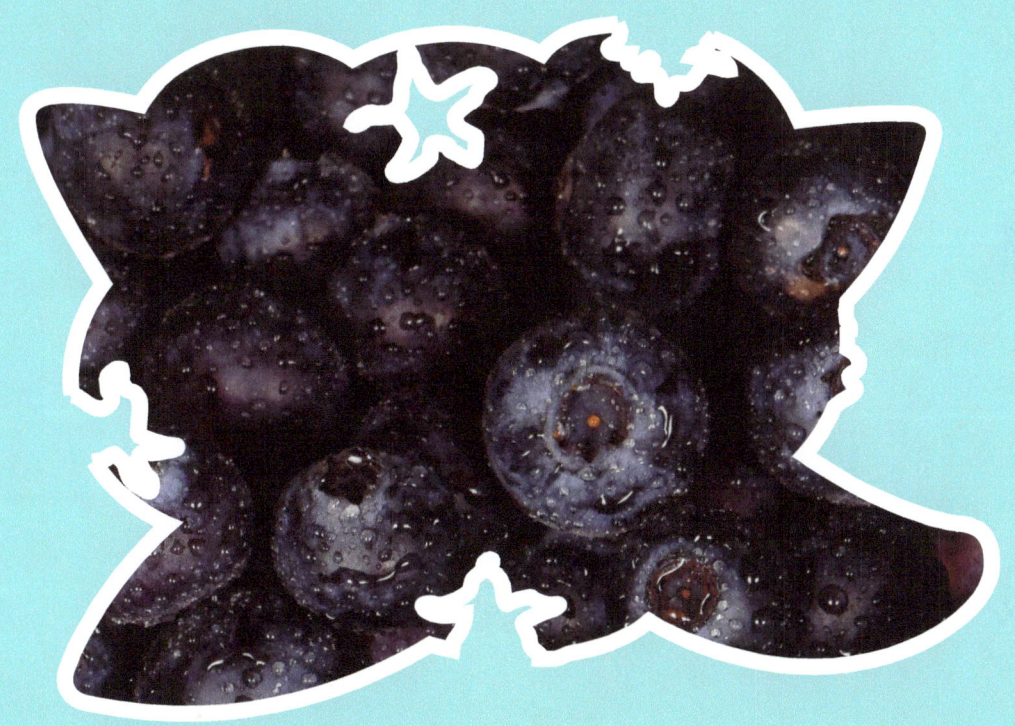

BLUEBERRIES

YELLOW

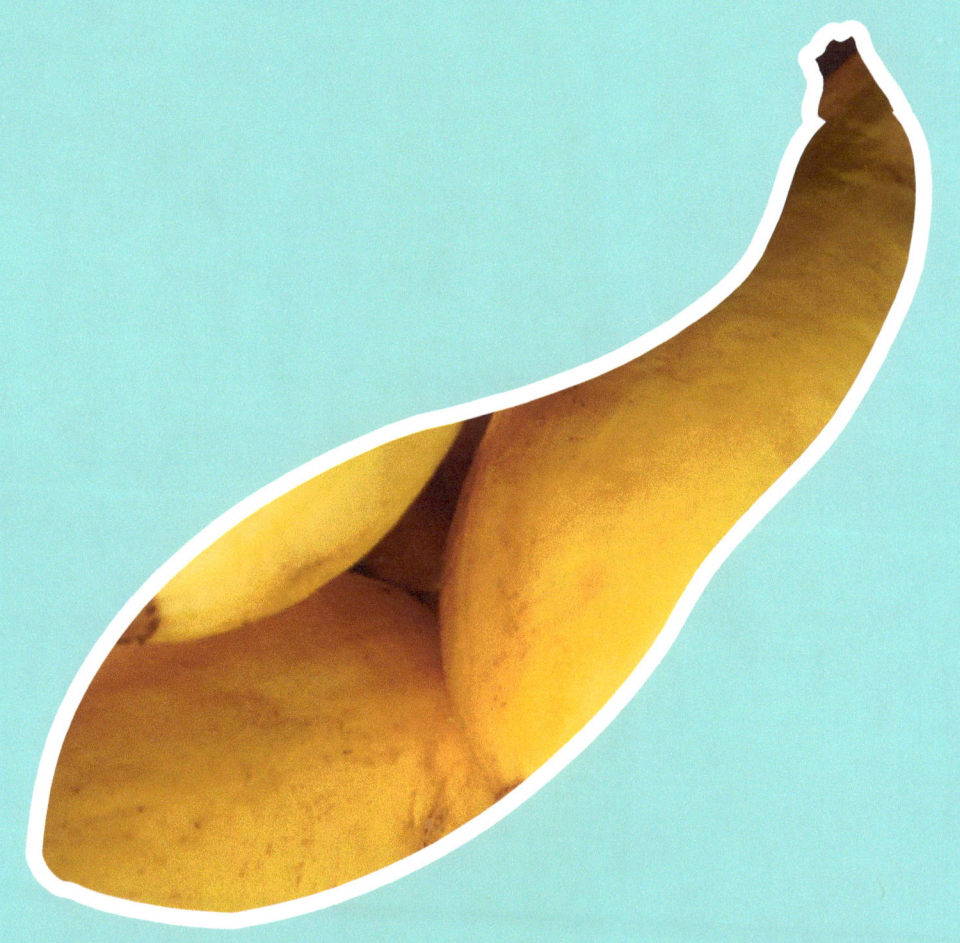

YELLOW SQUASH

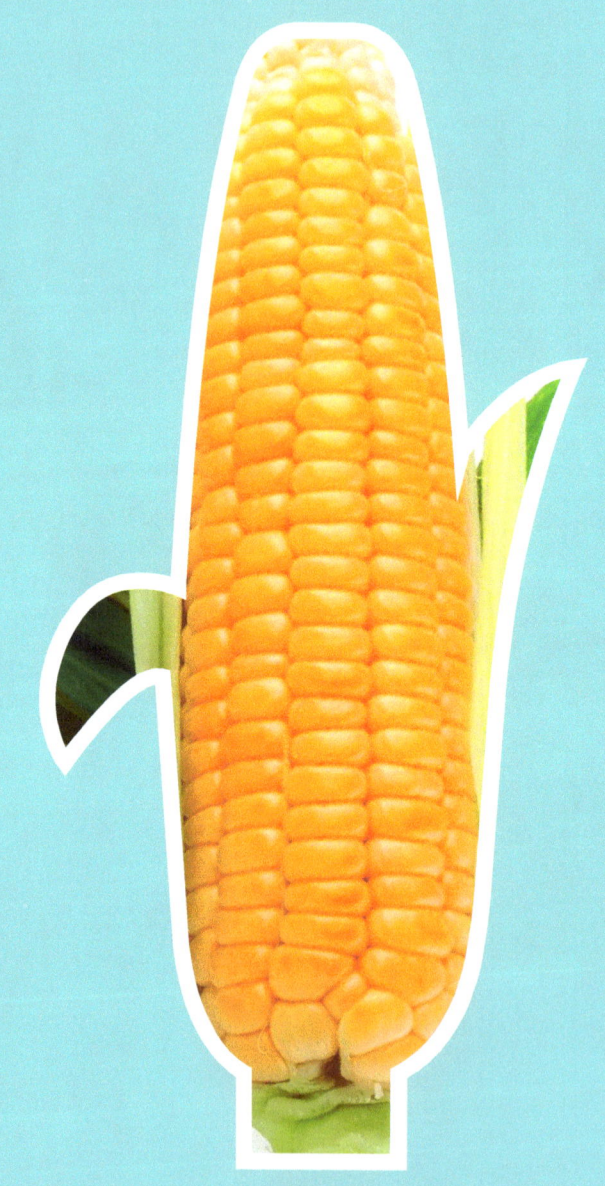

CORN

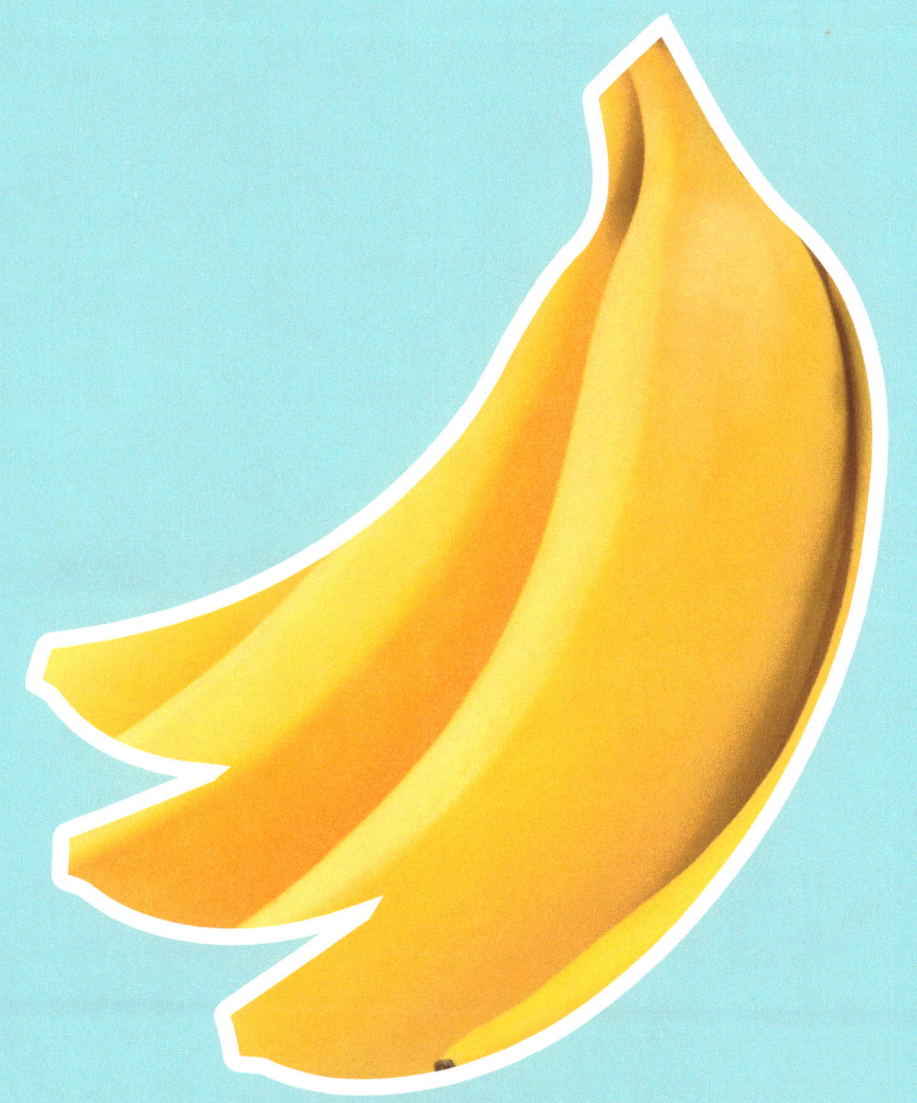

BANANAS

WHITE

ONIONS

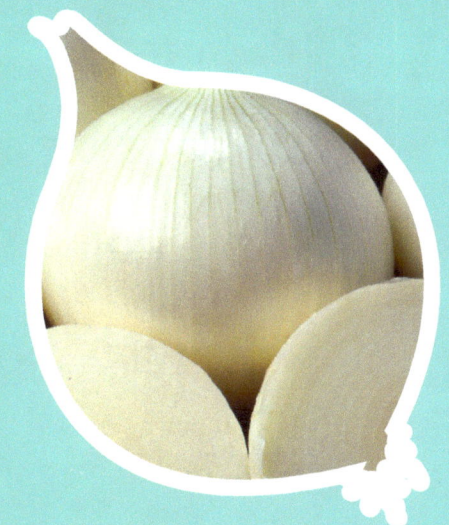

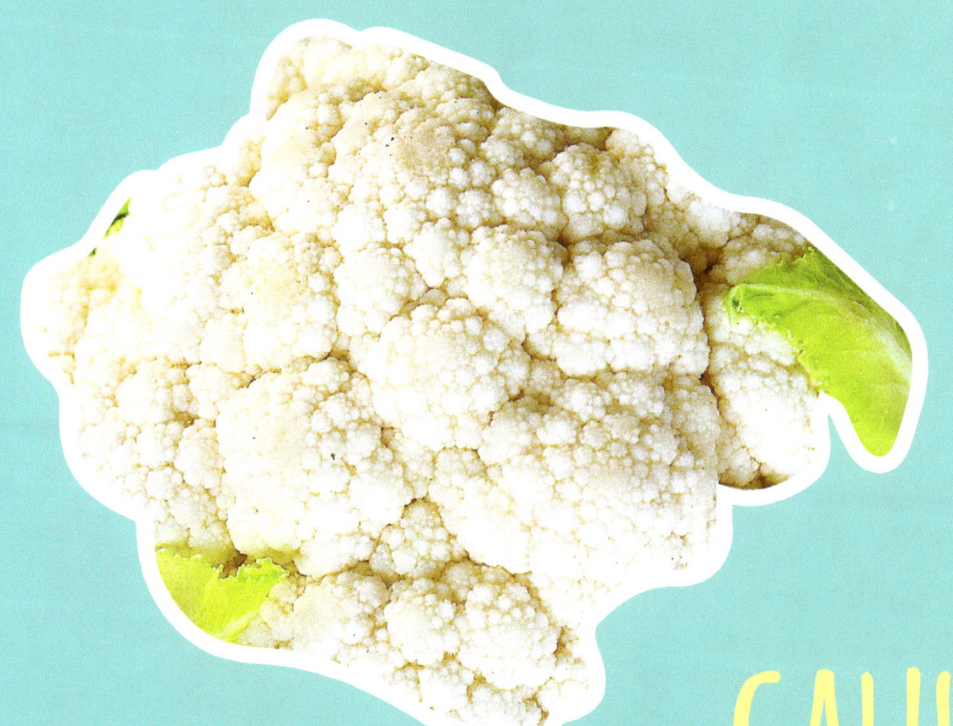

CAULIFLOWER

ORANGE

BELL PEPPERS

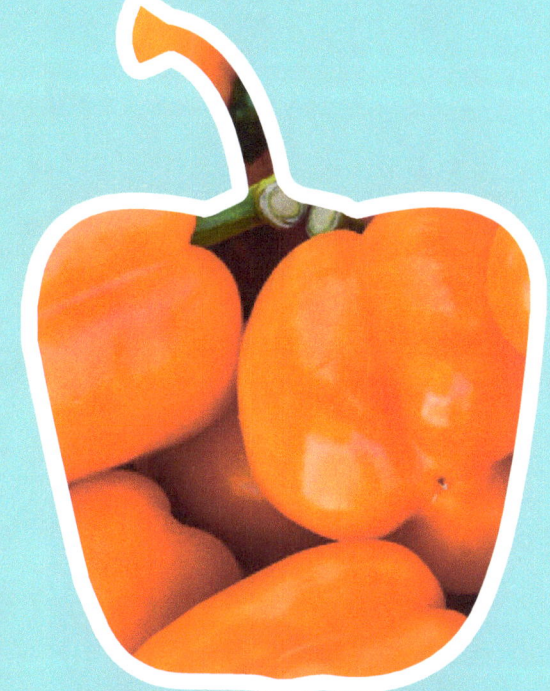

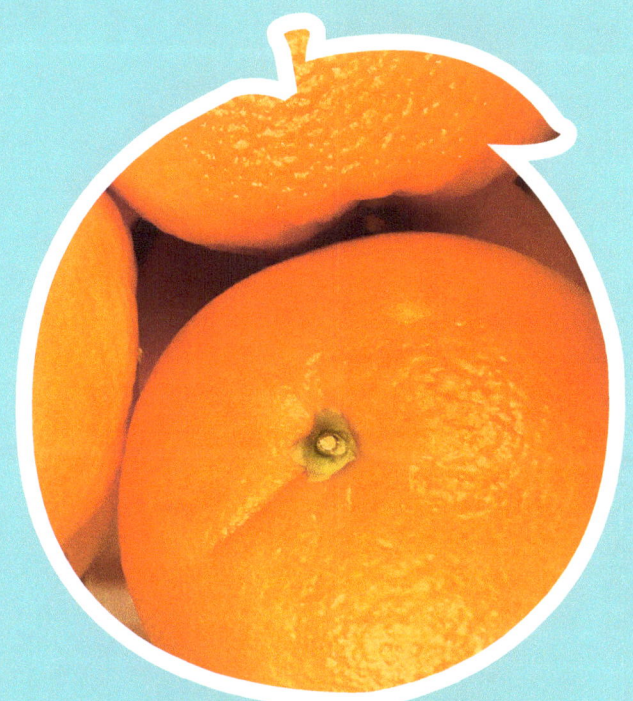

ORANGES

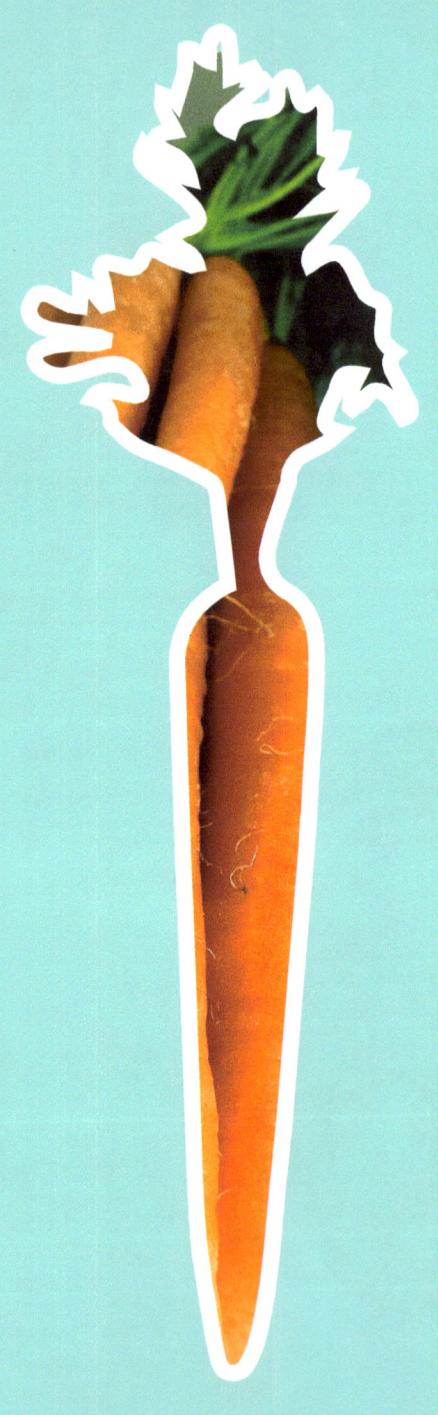

CARROTS

GREEN

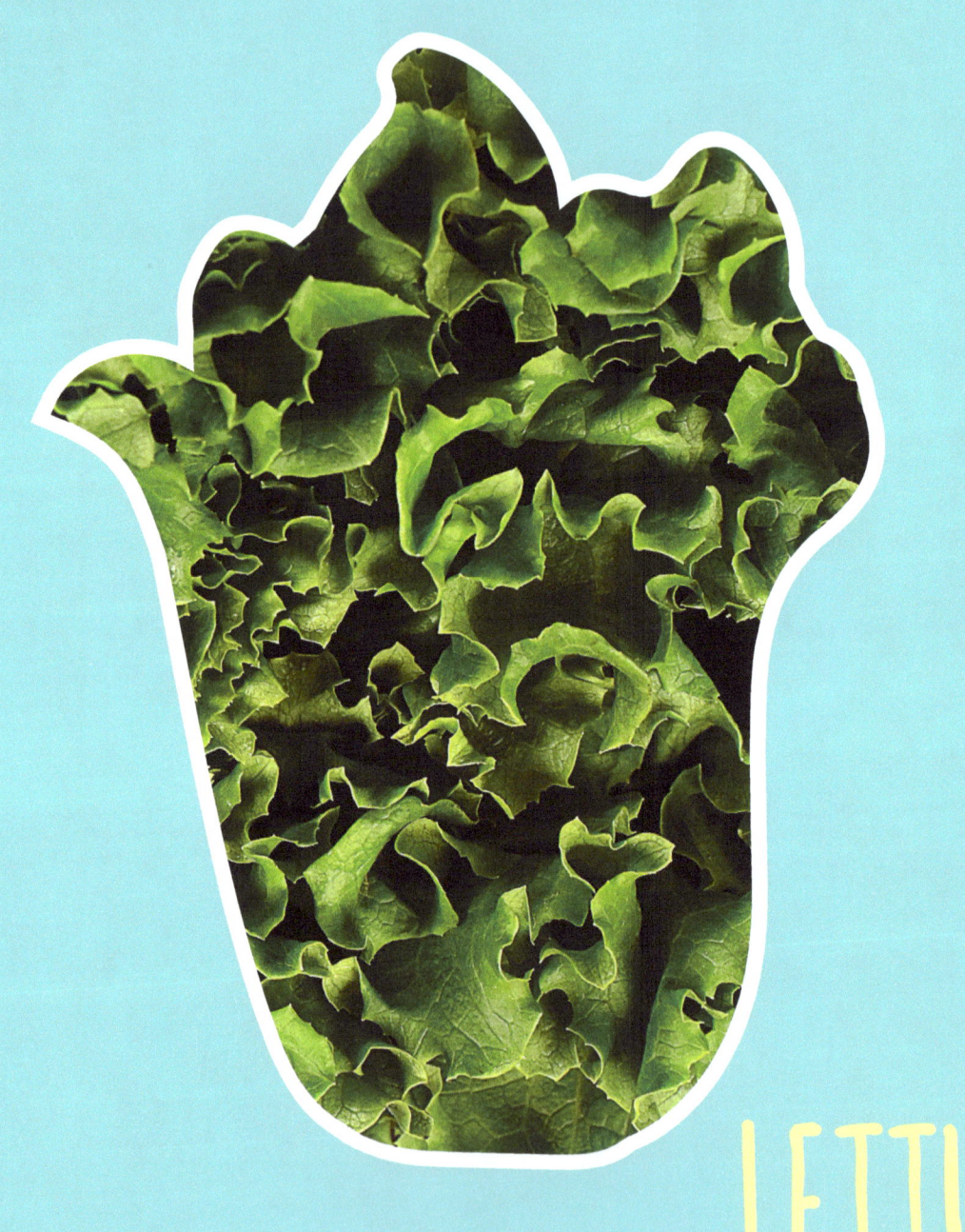

LETTUCE

GREEN BEANS

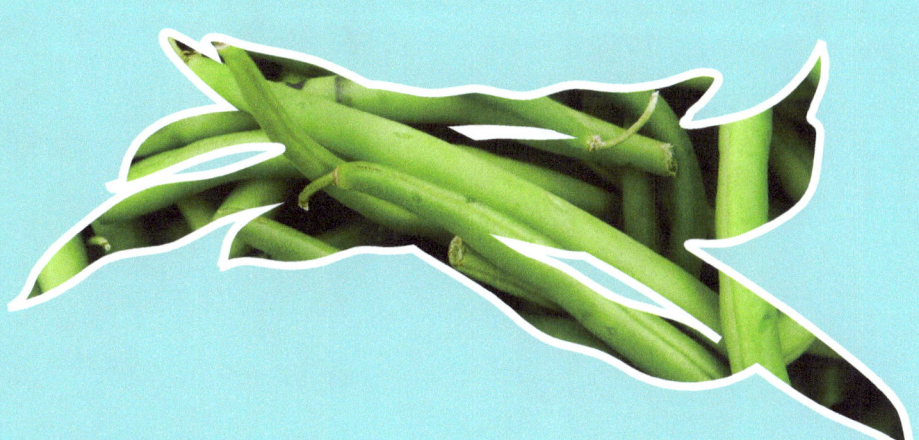

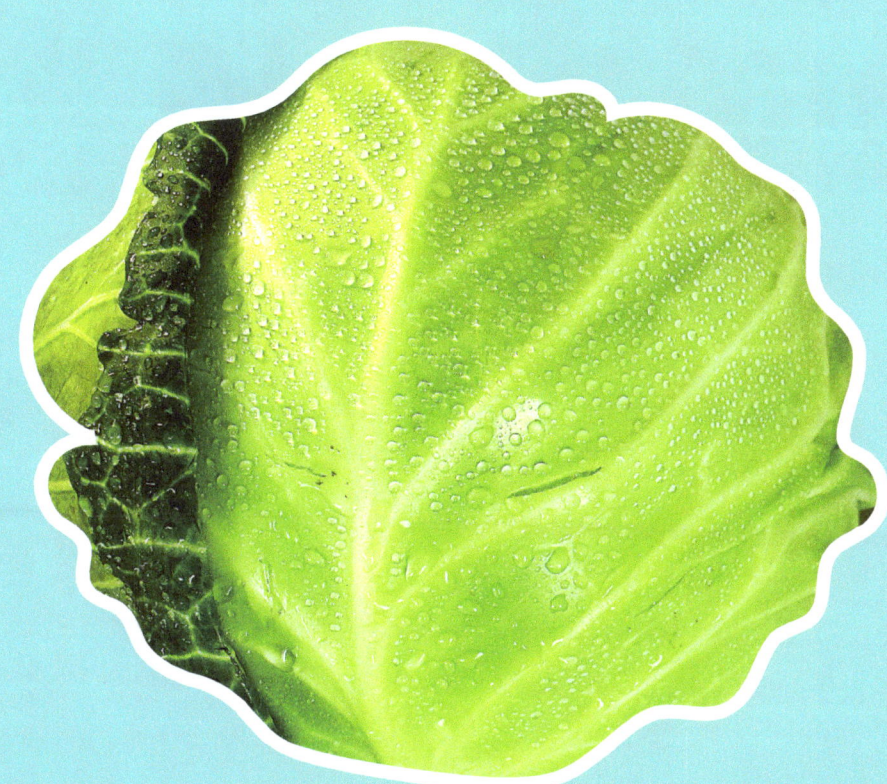

CABBAGE

APPLES

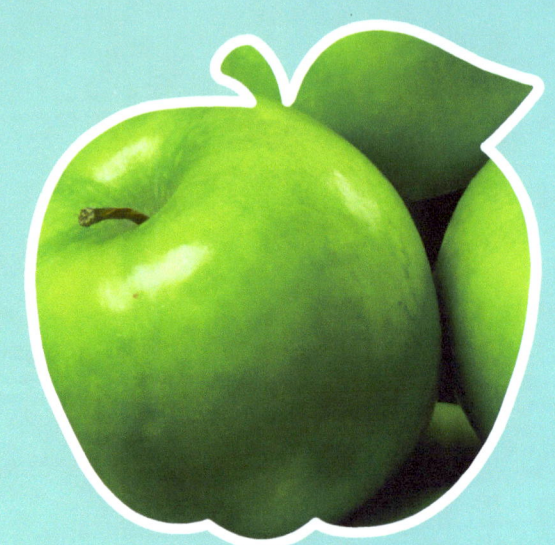

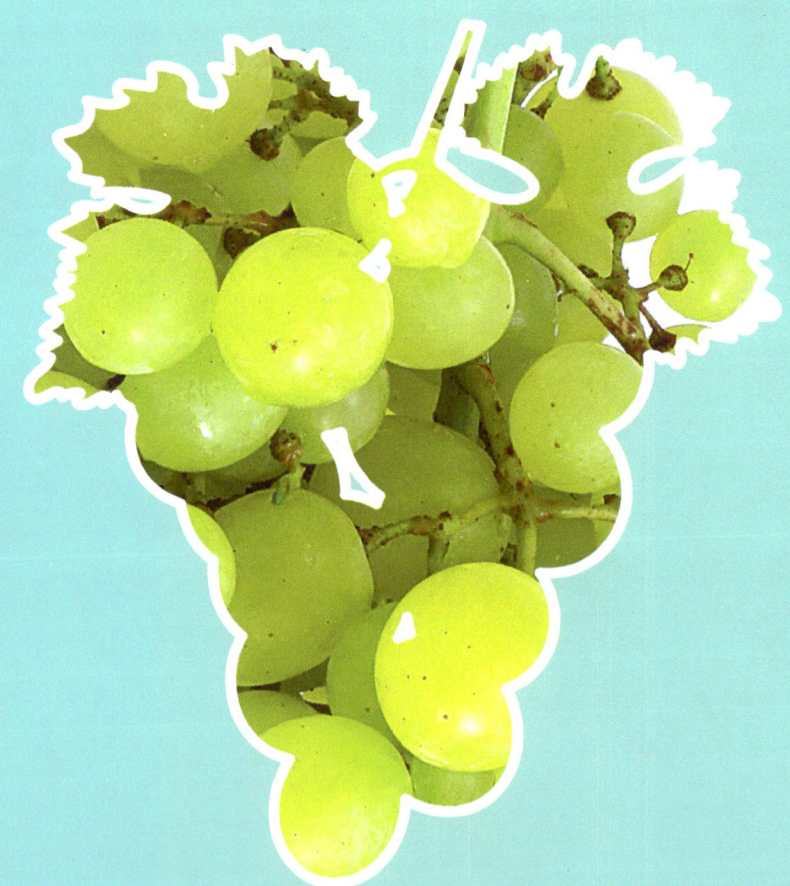

GRAPES

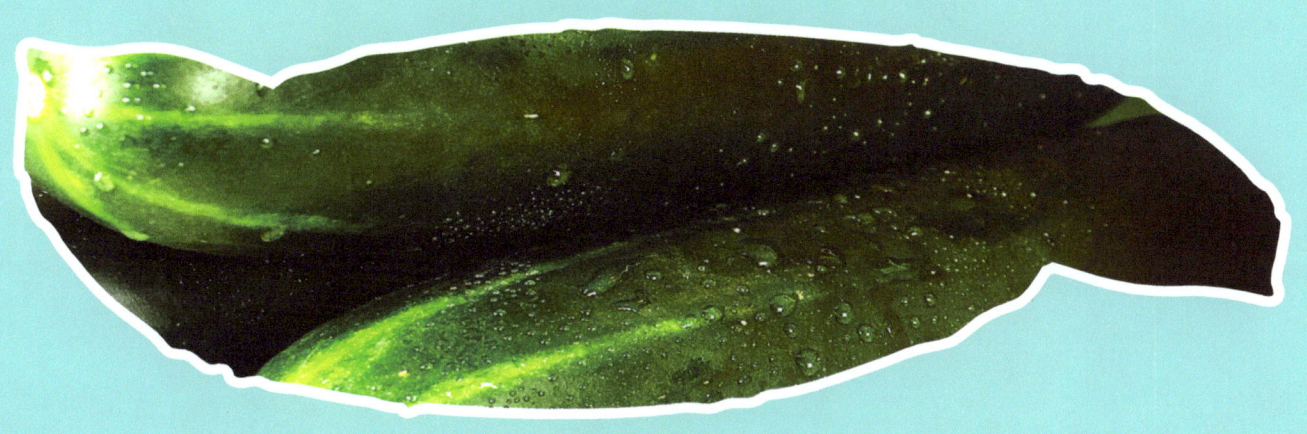

CUCUMBERS

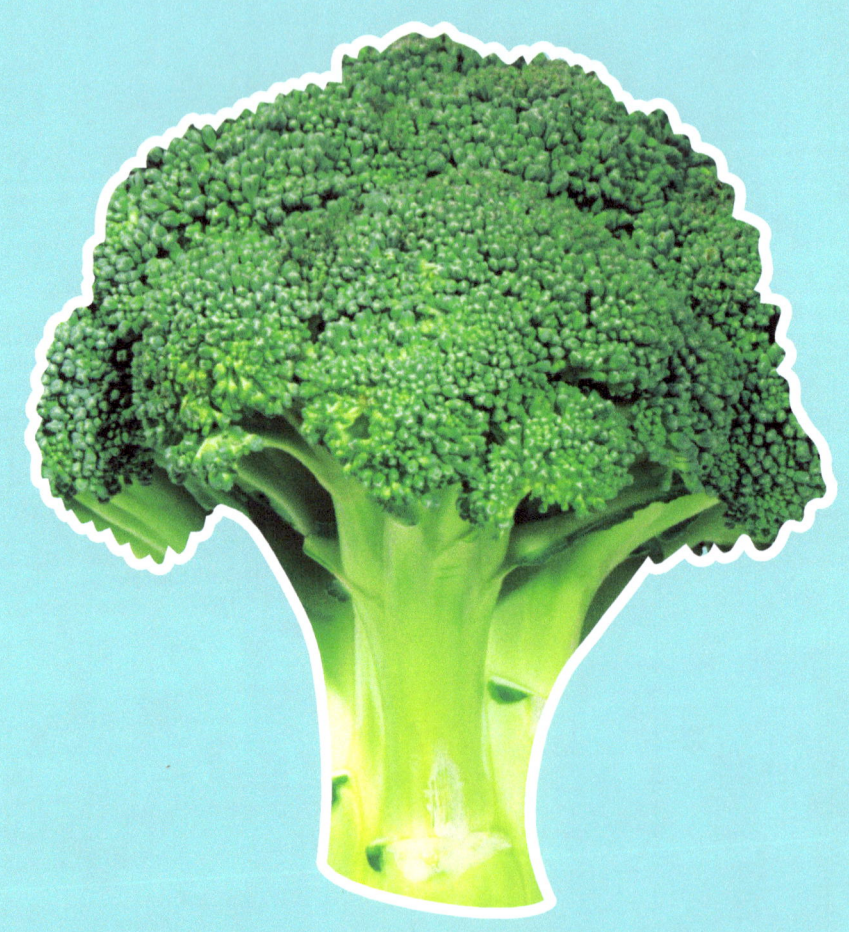

BROCCOLI

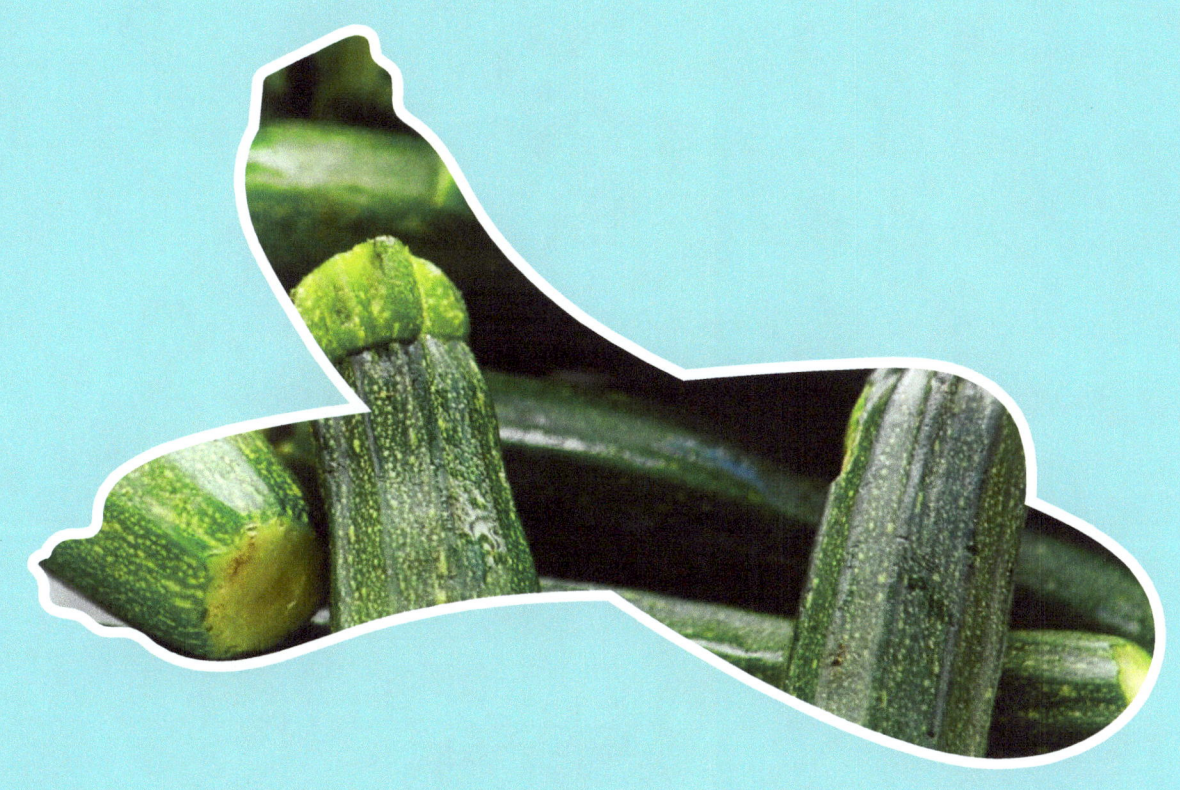

ZUCCHINI

AND

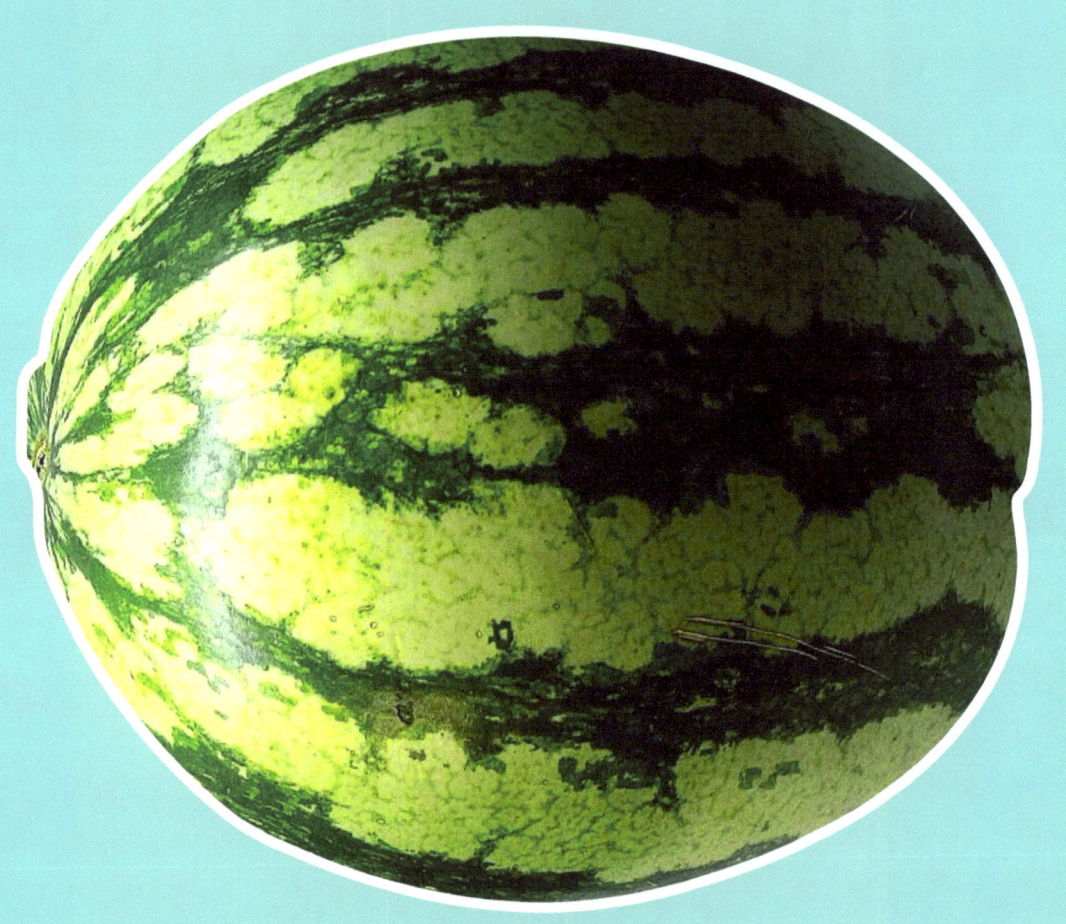

WATERMELON

WAIT!
WATERMELON
ISN'T
GREEN!
IT'S...

RED

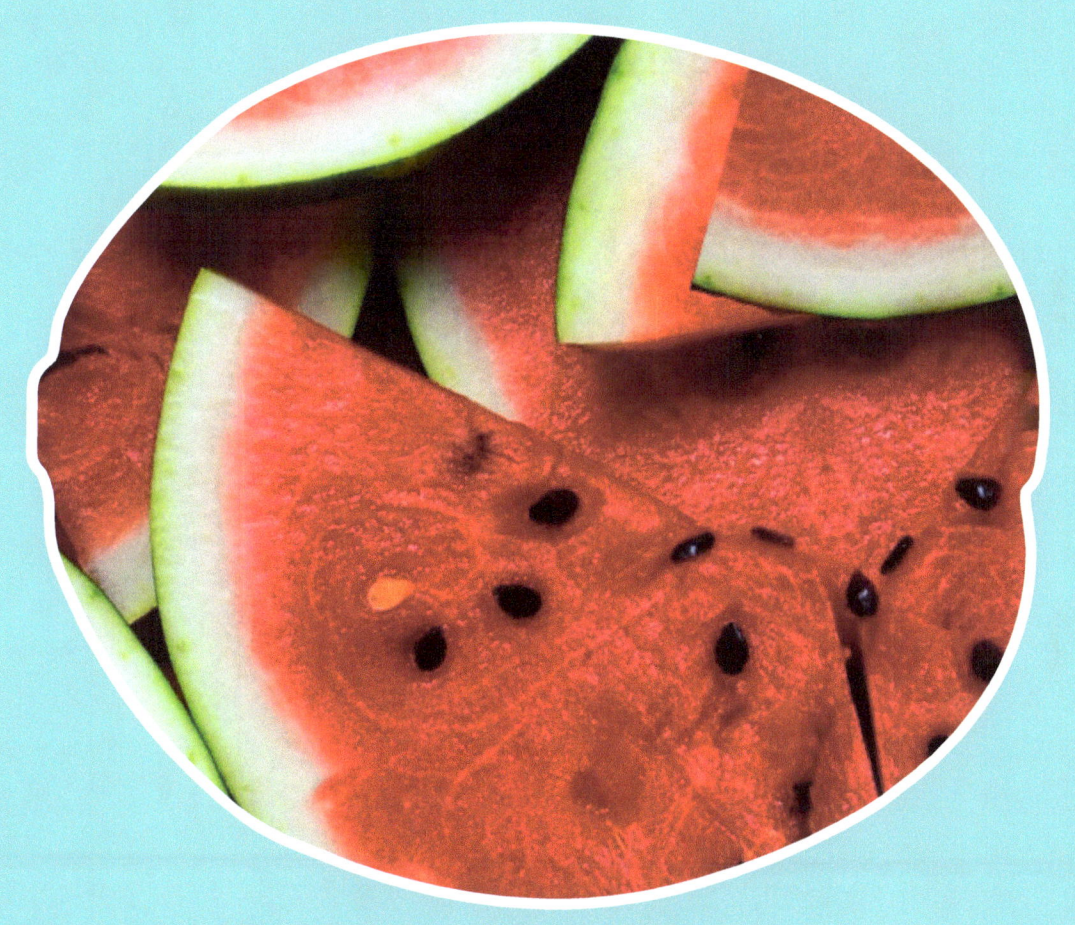

WATERMELON

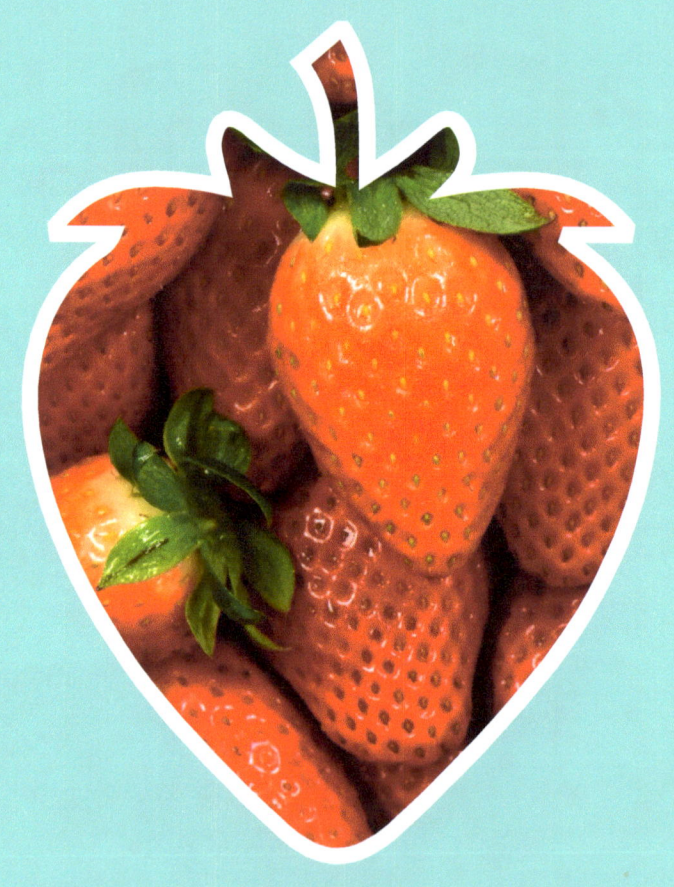

STRAWBERRIES

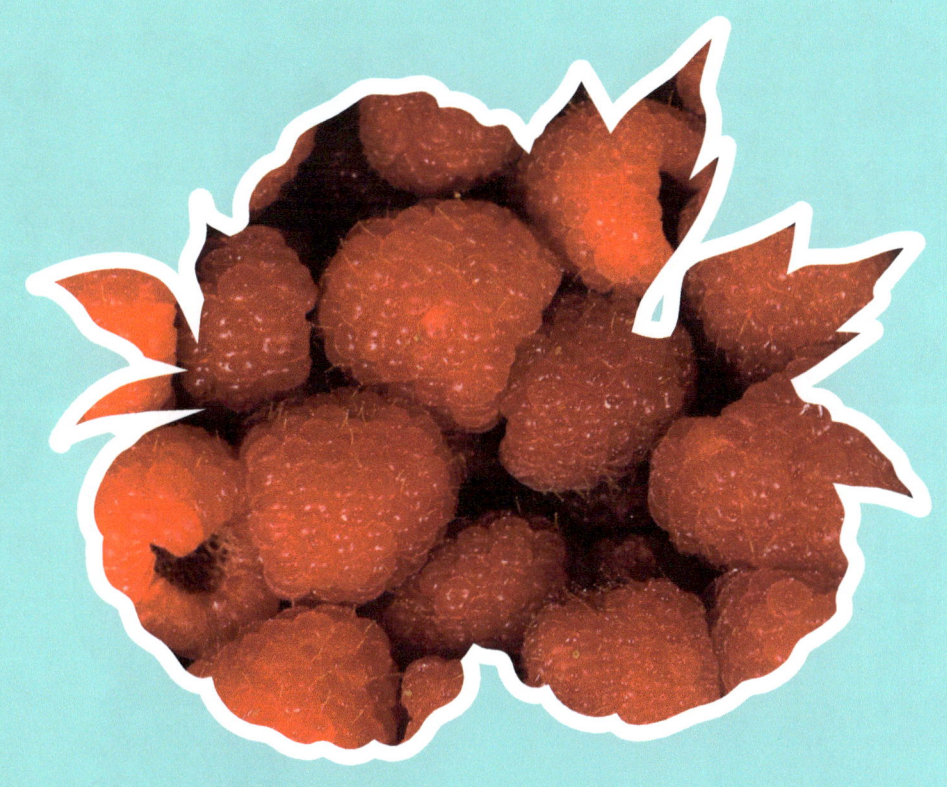

RASPBERRIES

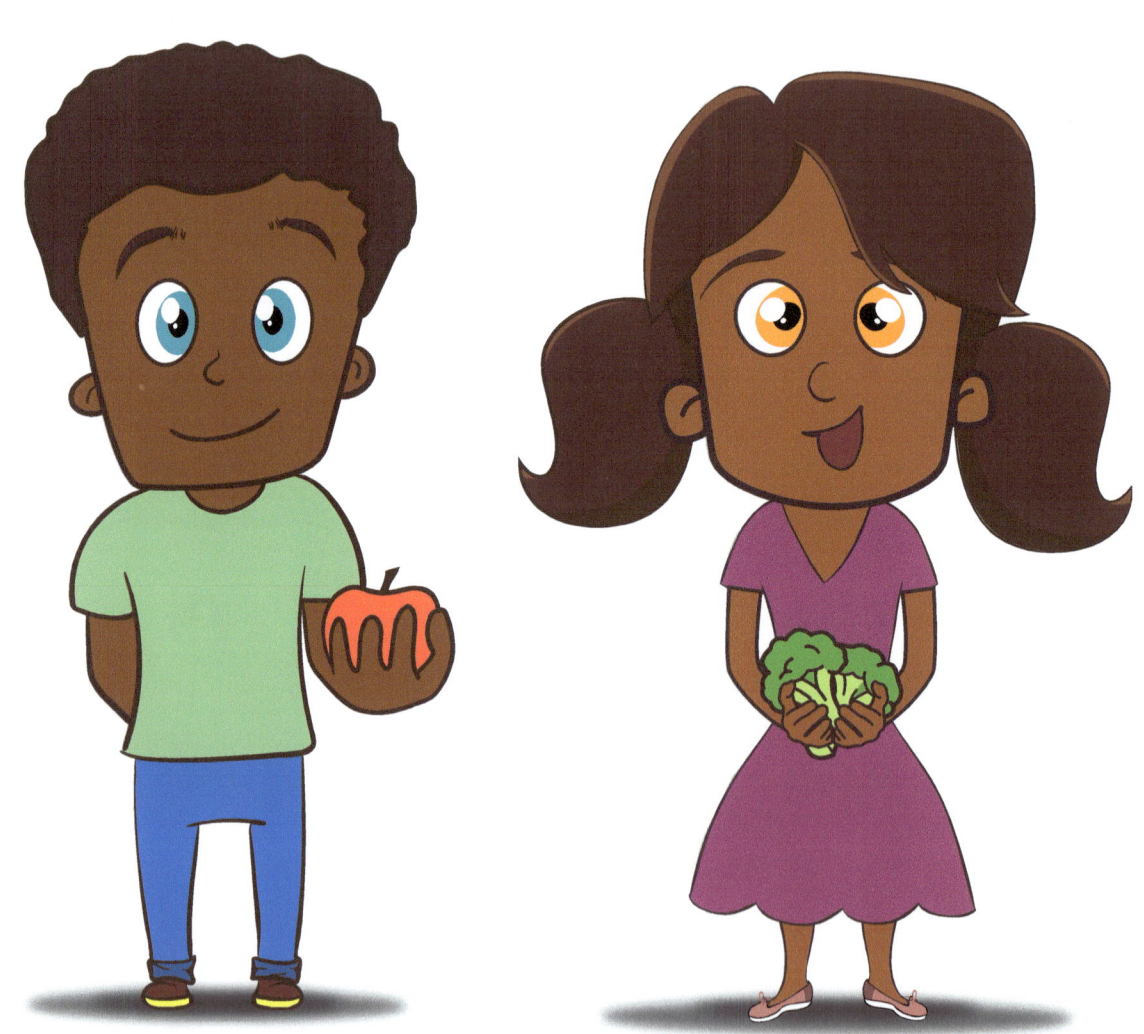

THESE VIVID COLORS IN OUR FRIDGE
ARE WHAT WE LOVE TO EAT.
YUMMY FRUITS
AND VEGETABLES
ARE OUR

FAVORITE,
DELECTABLE,
DELIGHTFUL,
NUTRITIOUS,
EVERY DAY,
TREMENDOUS

TREAT!

FOR EVERYONE, ESPECIALLY, PARENTS AND PRE-SCHOOL TEACHERS

Here are some activities that you can do to bring you, children and food together.

1. Make a grocery shopping list together!

2. Give each child a notepad and pen (young children can pretend to write and can still, verbally, help). Sit down with them, with your own notepad and pen, and make a list of what everyone wants to buy. Use this as an opportunity to point out healthy food from junk food, expensive foods from affordable foods and other wise shopping ideas.

3. Shop together!
With lists in hand, go grocery shopping. As you shop together, point out what item you are choosing to put in the basket and why, to you, it is a wise choice. Help children find what is on their list and allow them to place their items in the basket.
Children can help at checkout by taking items out of the basket. Even a young child, in the child seat of the cart can help place items onto the conveyor belt.

4. Carry groceries together!
Place light items in bags that children can handle.
Remind them how "many hands make light work"!

5. Wash fruits and vegetables together!
Talk about all the colors!

6. Prepare food together!
Give children a space to work that has easy clean-up.
Children can:
Cut (soft items with a bread knife), spread, smush, measure (with help), add ingredients, break eggs (with help), pour, stir or use an electric mixer (with help).

7. Cook food together!
Set up a step stool so children can watch you cook. Have, at most, 4 children at a time. Talk about fire/stove safety, pot holders, spatulas, woks, pots – whatever you are using can be named and explained. Talk about how wonderful everything smells!

8. Set the table together!
Talk about everything you are putting on the table and why and where you are putting it!

9. Enjoy eating together!
Strike up a great conversation as you eat!

10. Clean up together!
Children can:
Carry items they can handle from the table to the sink, throw garbage in the trash, compost and recycling bins, rinse items they can handle, help arrange dishes in the dishwasher, put in the soap and close the door!

By doing these everyday tasks together, you are creating, teaching and bonding with each child on a deep level. It is a level as deep as our primeval sense of smell, our absolute love of food and all the wonderful feelings that go with eating a meal!

EATING HEALTHY
MADE
EASY & SIMPLE

YES

FRUIT

Fresh or frozen fruit
Canned fruit   buy "packed in its own juices"
100% fruit juice   diluted by 50% water
Spritzers   sugar free
Fruit water

VEGETABLES

Fresh or frozen vegetables
Canned vegetables   buy low sodium, little or no sugar
Vegetable juice
Cucumber water

PROTEIN

Fresh or frozen meat,
fish, poultry
Canned   buy low sodium, little or no sugar
Lunchmeat   buy low sodium, little or no sugar
Nuts
Seeds
Beans   buy low sodium, little or no sugar
Grains/Breads   whole grains/ go Gluten-Free if
Seaweed   you choose
Mushrooms

DAIRY

All dairy products   moderate use
Alternative dairy
products

CONDIMENTS

Sea salt/ Iodized
Black Pepper
Margarine
Honey(not for children
under two), Agave Nectar,
Raw Sugar, Maple Syrup

Ketchup, Mustard,
Mayonnaise, Relish,
Pickles
Soy Sauce   buy low sodium
Salad Dressing   buy low sodium, little sugar
Spices
Tea
Coffee

WATER

As much as you want to drink!
eight, 8oz. glasses (8x8 rule)

NO   10% OF THE TIME OR LESS

Fast food
Fried food
Canned fruit
Canned vegetables   in heavy syrup
Lunchmeat   high in sodium and sugar
Regular Salt   high in sodium and sugar
White Sugar
Corn Syrup
Soda
Power Drinks
White bread
Food coloring
MSG (monosodium glutamate)
Nitrates
Any ingredients that you can't
pronounce or haven't researched

IF AND WHEN POSSIBLE, BUY FOOD THAT IS:

Organic   (try your local Farmer's Market)
Free running/grazing
No hormones
Non GMO
No antibiotics

ABOUT THE AUTHOR

Mariah Debra Gale Messinger is the mother of boy/girl twins.

In her travels, she has lived in Central New Jersey, Washington DC, the Blue Ridge Mountains of Virginia, Santa Cruz, CA, the wilderness of Wolf Creek, OR and, then, finally settled in San Francisco

It was in Afton, VA in the Blue Ridge Mountains, that she began writing and illustrating children's books. First, for her twin's delight and, then, because the stories would not stop coming out of her! At this time, Mariah is Owner/Director/Head Teacher of a home based Pre-school, Pre-K, Daycare. Children are and have always been an integral part of her life. This book was inspired by her own experience, albeit just one of many...

For more of Mariah's Children's Books, visit Mariah's website:

www.mariahdebragalemessinger.com

For more insights into children visit Mariah's daughter Jenn's website:

www.jennieve.ca

MORE BOOKS BY THIS AUTHOR

Upon a Pillow
The Balloon Man
Wisteria's Candle
Potty Poems

By this author and illustrated by Jennieve Consalvo

The Wind In This City
The Sprites Went Out To Play!
Where Is It? Where Can It Be?